Mohamed Zairi
Mohamed Nabil Nessib

Biomechanics of Superior Femoral Epiphysis in Adolescents

Mohamed Zairi
Mohamed Nabil Nessib

Biomechanics of Superior Femoral Epiphysis in Adolescents

Risk Factors and Stability Criteria

ScienciaScripts

Imprint

Any brand names and product names mentioned in this book are subject to trademark, brand or patent protection and are trademarks or registered trademarks of their respective holders. The use of brand names, product names, common names, trade names, product descriptions etc. even without a particular marking in this work is in no way to be construed to mean that such names may be regarded as unrestricted in respect of trademark and brand protection legislation and could thus be used by anyone.

Cover image: www.ingimage.com

This book is a translation from the original published under ISBN 978-620-3-44154-3.

Publisher:
Sciencia Scripts
is a trademark of
Dodo Books Indian Ocean Ltd. and OmniScriptum S.R.L Publishing group
Str. Armeneasca 28/1, office 1, Chisinau MD-2012, Republic of Moldova, Europe
Printed at: see last page
ISBN: 978-620-5-25550-6

BIOMECHANICS FROM FEMORAL EPIPHYSIOLYSIS SUPERIOR AT THE ADOLESCENT: RISK FACTORS AND STABILITY CRITERIA

TABLE OF CONTENTS

INTRODUCTION

In order to understand the natural history of upper femoral epiphysiolysis (UFE), it is essential to study its components, its evolution and its consequences [1]. It is acceptec that the epiphysis slips in relation to the femoral neck, whereas in reality it is the neck that slips in relation to the epiphysis, which is attached to the acetabulum by the round ligament. This displacement occurs through the basicapital growth plate and precisely at the level of the pathological hypertrophic layer. The ethiopathogenesis is not yet elucidated but several risk factors have been suggested. The main risk factor is overweight. Other metabolic factors have been incriminated such as hypothyroidism, growth hormone deficiency and chronic renal faiiure. The common denominator between all these risk factors is the decreased biomechanical strength of the subcapital growth plate and its perichondral shell. Percutaneous screw fixation, with or without reduction, is the gold standard for the management of small and medium displacement PSA. The objectives of our work were to:

1. Identify the biomechanical factors involved in the occurrence of epiphysiolysis femoral through a case series and a review of the literature.
2. To study the biomechanical factors of stability of the upper femoral epiphysis after percutaneous screw fixation allowing healing without sequelae.

METHODS

1. Type of the study

This is a retrospective, single-center, longitudinal study of 76 patients, 7 of whom presented with a bilateral form; that is, 83 hips treated for EFS by percutaneous screw fixation in the department of orthopedics f o r children and adolescents at the Béchir Hamza Hospital in Tunis over a period of seven years from January 1, 2013, to December 31, 2019. Our mean recoil was 5.66 years with extremes ranging from 1.33 years to 7.58 years.

2. Population of the study

2.1. Criteria for inclusion

We included in our study:

- EFS treated exclusively by percutaneous screwing.

- A postoperative follow-up of at least 12 months.

2.2. Criteria for exclusion

Patients who had postoperative support before 6 weeks were excluded.

2.3. Non-inclusion criteria

The non-inclusion criterion was EFS treated by open reduction.

3. Methods

3.1. Collection of data

Epidemiological, clinical, radiological, therapeutic and evolutionary data of each patient were collected from the medical records. The data were processed using Excel software.

3.2. Analysis statistics

The statistical analysis of the data collected was carried out using the software SPSS version 24.

3.3. Research bibliography

The literature search was performed using the following search engines: Science Direct, Pubmed, Cochrane, and Google Scholer.

3.4. Variants and classifications (Appendices 1-4)

In our study, we used three types of classification and one score.
- Fahey and O'Brien's classification [2] which divides EFS according to the duration of symptoms.

- Classification of Loder and Kallio that judges the stability of EFS [3,4].
- Southwick's radiographic classification that divides EFS according to the tilt angle [5].

- Postel and Merle d'Aubigné scoring (PMA) which allows the evaluation of the results of the surgery [6].

RESULTS

1. Data epidemiological

1.1. Distribution by gender

Our study included 76 patients, 53 of whom were boys (69.7%) and 23 girls (30.3%). There was a clear male predominance with a sex ratio of 2.3.

1.2. Distribution by age

Age at surgery ranged from 9 to 16 years with an average of 12.5 years.

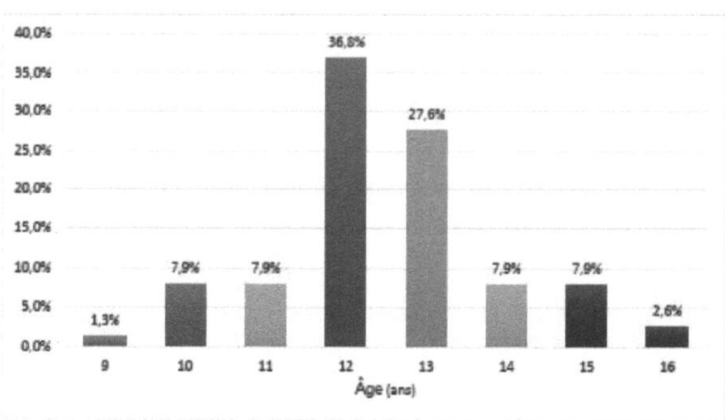

Figure 1: Age distribution.

1.3. Weight and morphotype

58% of the cases (44 patients) had a weight > +3 SD (Standard Deviations) of which 11% (8 patients) had an adiposogenic morphotype, 13% of the cases (10 patients) had a weight between +2 and +3 SD and 29% (22 patients) had a normal weight.

1.4. Notion of trauma

Trauma was found in 35.5% of cases, i.e., in 27 patients. In most cases, it was minimal, following a fall from a height.

1.5. Time to take charge

The delay between EFS diagnosis and surgical management did not exceed 24 hours for all patients except one who was operated on after 7 days in connection with an anesthetic contraindication.

2. Data clinical

2.1. Start of the symptomatology

The onset was acute in 22.9% of patients (19 hips). It was chronic in 60.2% (50 hips) and acute on a chronic background in 16.9% (14 hips).

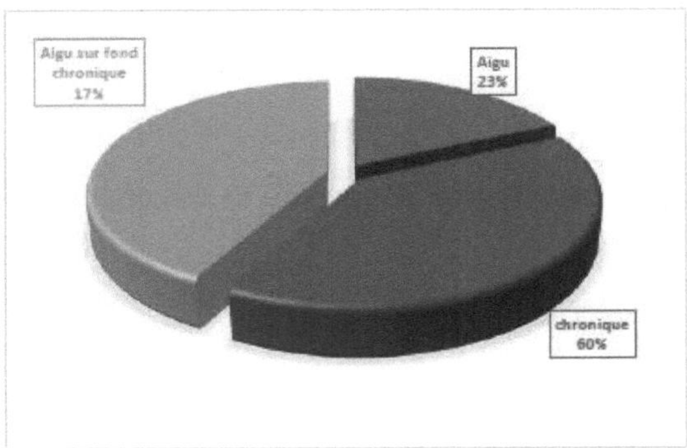

Figure 2: Distribution according to mode of onset.

2.2. Notion of stability

In our series, the stable form represented 60% (50 hips) and the unstable form 40% (33 hips).

2.3. On the side reached

Among the 76 patients operated on, 7 presented a bilateral form, i.e. 9.2%. of cases.EFS was unilateral in 90.8% of cases, i.e. 69 patients. The left side was the most affected with 59.2% of cases.

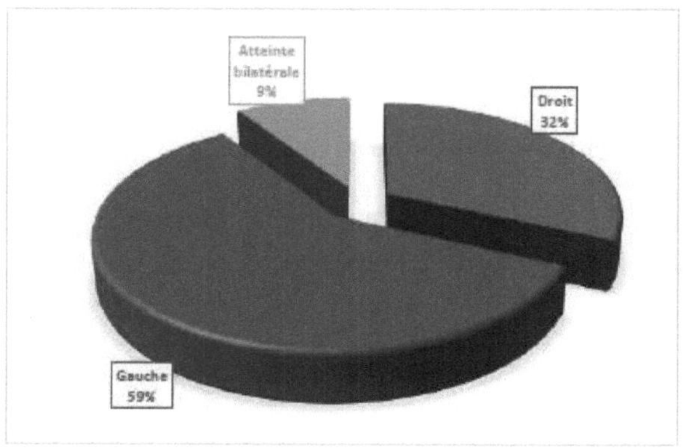

Figure 3: Distribution according to the affected side.

2.4. Signs clinical

2.4.1. Signs functional

Lameness was the main reason for consultation of the patients. It concerned 67 hips out of 83, i.e. a percentage of 88.1%. Table I below shows the distribution of functional signs in our patients.

Table I: Distribution of functional signs in our patients.

Functional sign	Patients	Percentage
Lameness	67	88,1%
Inguinal pain	23	30,2%
Partial functional impotence	21	27,6%
Total functional impotence	30	39,4%
Isolated gonalgia	17	22,3%

2.4.2. Signs physical

Internal rotation limitation, decreased abduction, and external rotation walking were the most common physical signs found on clinical examination.Table II shows the distribution of physical signs in our patients.

Table II: Distribution of physical signs in our patients.

Physical sign	Hips	Percentage
Limitation of internal rotation	80	96%
Decreased abduction	74	89%
Walking in external rotation	32	38,5%
Positive Drehmann sign	10	12%
Amyotrophy of the thigh	21	25,3%

3. X-ray of the pelvis from the front and the hips from the side (Lauenstein Incidence)

Confirm the positive diagnosis and classify the trip. We calculated the tilt angle according to Southwick's method and according to In the latter, the EFS were classified into three stages. For the 83 hips studied, we obtained:

- Stage I: 47% (39 hips)

- Stage II: 43.3% (36 hips)

- Stage III: 9.7% (08 hips)

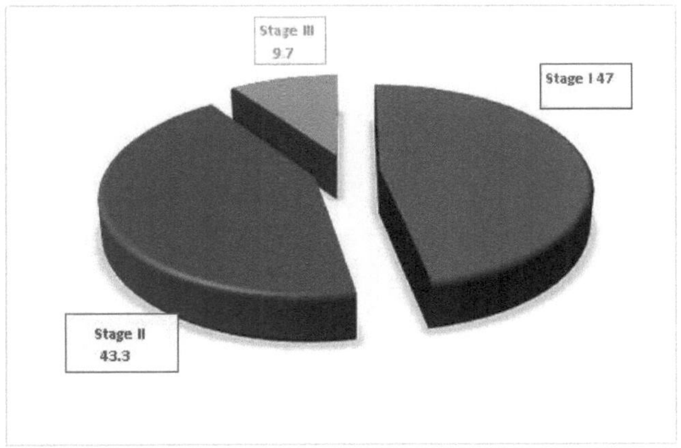

Figure 4: Distribution by EFS stage.

4. Treatment

4.1. Landfill of the member

From the moment of hospitalization, all our patients were put under traction until the the screwing process.

4.2. Reduction before screwing

In our series, 56.6% of the cases (47 hips) were fixed without any reduction and 43.4% of the cases (36 hips) were fixed after gentle and partial reduction.

4.3. Means of fixation

For the fixation of the epiphysis, we used a Veet-Woot type screw, with washer, designed and manufactured in Tunisia. It is a Titanium screw, cannulated, with full thread and self-tapping. It has a large head and measures 7.0 mm in diameter (Figure 5).

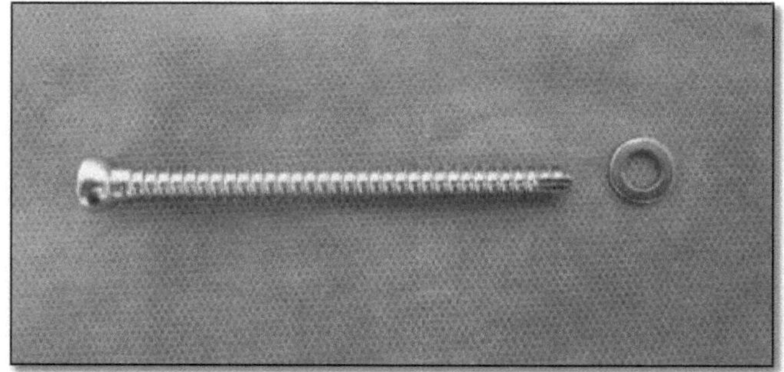

Figure 5: Cannulated screw with washer used in epiphysis fixation during EFS in the pediatric orthopedic department at the Béchir Hamza Hospital in Tunis.

4.4. Percutaneous screwing : Figure 6 and 7

Also known as cervicocephalic osteosynthesis, percutaneous screwing is to prevent the continuation of the slide or to prevent its occurrence.
In our series, we operated on 76 patients, 7 of whom had a bilateral form in whom bilateral percutaneous screw fixation was decided upon immediately, i.e., 9% of the cases.
For the 69 patients with a unilateral form, 71% of the cases had a unilateral percutaneous screw fixation (49 patients) and 29% had, in addition, a contralateral prophylactic percutaneous screw fixation of the hip deemed healthy (20 patients). The screw was inserted with the aid of a guide pin and preparation of the path with a drill and then an auger. An attempt was always made to have the epiphyseal cap held at its center on the front and side views. At least three turns of coils should hold the cap.

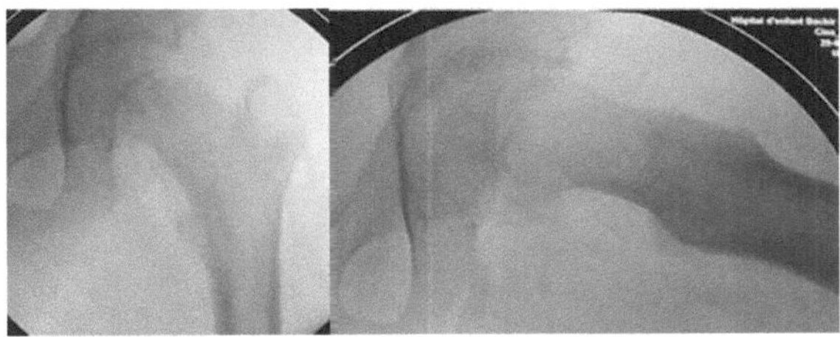

Figure 6: Reduced stage II EFS: a residual displacement of 15° remains.

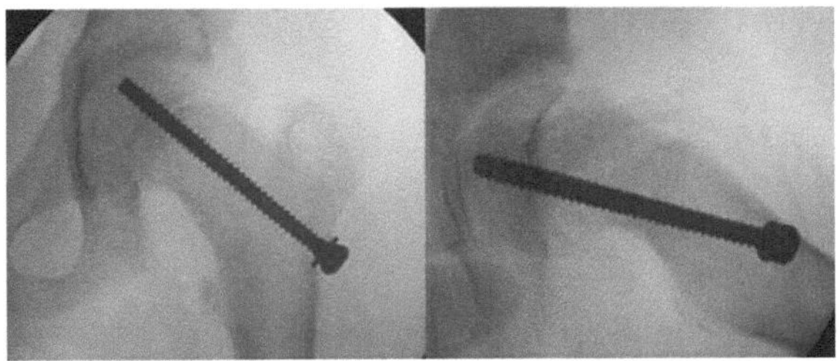

Figure 7: Percutaneous screwing, the screw is in the center of the cap from the front and from the side and at least three turns of the thread in the cap for better stability.

4.5. Postoperative radiography immediate

It allows us to check that the screw is well positioned and to calculate the residual tilt.

4.6. Unloading of the limb in postoperative

The strict ban on postoperative weight-bearing is 6 weeks for all patients.

5. Follow-up

We have constructed the tilt angle according to Southwick's method on

all of our patients' profile hip radiographs to determine residual tilt and deduce how many cases had progression of slip after screw fixation. We found that slip continued to progress significantly (>5°) in only one patient. It increased from 30° to 48°.

6. Evolution

6.1. Time to resume normal activity

The time to return to normal activity varied from 3 months to 1 year. 93.4% (71 patients) returned to normal activity within the first three months after screwing, 5.3% of cases (4 patients) between 4 and 6 months and 1.2% (1 patient)
at 1 year.

6.2. Time to resume schooling

The resumption of schooling was rapid for most of our patients. Its delay varied from 7 to 20 days with an average of 10 days.

6.4. Time limit for resuming an activity

In our department, we recommend stopping sports activities for at least at least 1 year to all children operated on by an EFS. The deadline of recovery of an activity sports activity inour series avaried from 1 to 2 years. 77.6% (59 patients) of the cases stopped sport for one year, 8% (6 patients) resumed after 2 years (11 patients) and 14.4% never resumed sport after screwing due to apprehension.

7. Evaluation of results

We evaluated the results of screwing based on the Postel and Merle d'Aubigné (PMA) scoring.At an average follow-up of 5.66 years, we obtained excellent results in 56.6% of cases, good results in 36.1%, fair results in 4.8% and poor results in 2.4% of cases.The results obtained according to the severity of the initial slip were:
- Stage I: 79.5% excellent, 18% good, no average results and only 1 bad result.

- Stage II: 38.9% excellent, 58.3% good, 2.8% average and no poor results.

- Stage III: 25% excellent, 25% good, 37.5% average and 12.5% poor results.

Tables III, IV and V below summarize our results.

Table III: Overall functional results after screw fixation according to PMA score.

Appreciation	Number of hips	Percentage
Excellent	47	56,6%
Coupons	30	36,1%
Means	4	4,8%
Bad	2	2,4%

Table IV: Screwing results according to the severity of the displacement.

a- In number of hips operated:

Results / Stadium	I	II	III	Total
Excellent	31	14	2	47
Coupons	7	21	2	30
Means	0	1	3	4
Bad	1	0	1	2
Total	39	36	8	83

b- In percentages:

Results / Stadium	I	II	III
Excellent	79,5%	38,9%	25%
Coupons	18%	58,3%	25%
Means	0%	2,8%	37,5%
Bad	2,5%	0%	12,5%

Table V: Screwing results according to the treatment.

a- In number of hips operated:

Treatment / Results	Excellent	Coupons	Means	Poor	Total
In situ screwing	29	18	0	0	47
Reduction + screwing	18	12	4	2	36
Total	47	30	4	2	83

b- In percentages:

Treatment / Results	Excellent	Coupons	Means	Bad
In situ screwing	61,7%	60%	0%	0%
Reduction + screwing	38,3%	40%	100%	100%

DISCUSSION

1. Etiopathogeny

The exact ethiopathogenesis of EFS is to date unknown. It is probably multifactorial [7]. Mechanical, endocrine and genetic factors as well as radio-chemotherapy seem to be involved in its genesis.

1.1. Factors mechanical

Three mechanical factors have been identified: obesity-related decrease in femoral anteversion, increased shear forces, and more recently the shape of the growth plate. Femoral anteversion is 9.8° in children with EFS while it is 25° in children without epiphysiolysis [8]. Obesity increases the forces applied to the upper end of the femur. This leads to excessive neck remodeling and decreases femoral anteversion [9]. The precise mechanism is still unknown. The weight of the subject and the action of the muscles exert forces in the frontal plane perpendicular to the plane of the upper femoral growth plate, corresponding to a compressive stress [10].

Because of the inclination and physiological anteversion of the neck, the supporting hip automatically flexes when the step is taken. The flexion will progressively eliminate the anteversion and put this supporting hip in functional retroversion. This mechanism is more important during fast walking and running (Figure 8).

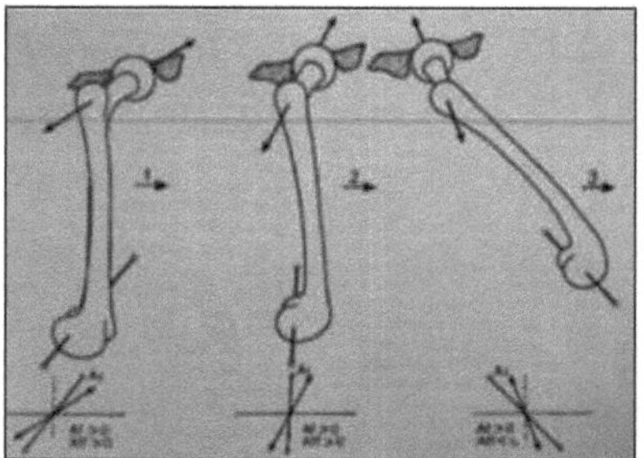

Figure 8: Hip flexion during rapid walking.
Transformation of anatomical anteversion into functional retroversion
[11].

The resultant force on the growth plate is anteroposterior in the horizontal plane. It is composed of a KK' component in the axis of the neck, maintaining head-neck cohesion, and a KS component directed posteriorly against the posterior edge of the acetabulum. The greater the anatomical or functional retroversion, the more the cohesion component decreases and the more the shear stress increases (Figure 9).

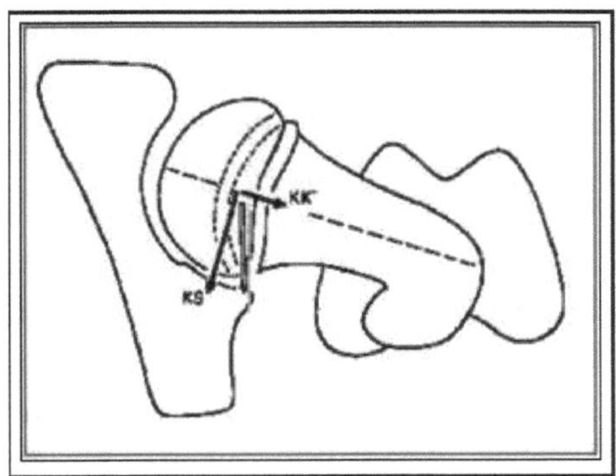

**Figure 9: Decomposition of the anteroposterior stress experienced by the femoral epiphysis in a horizontal plane into two components: a head-neck cohesion component KK
and a shear component KS [11].**

Also in favor of a mechanical explanation, it has been shown that the risk of epiphysiolysis was greater in children with a greater slope of the upper femoral growth plate (perpendicular to the axis of the femoral neck) as shown in Figure 10 below on the right image [12].

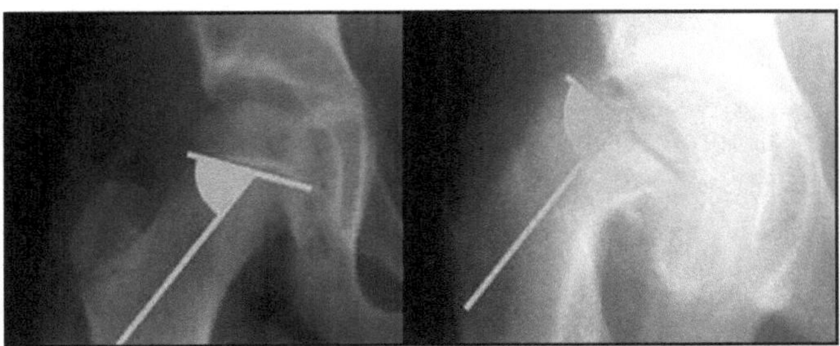

Figure 10: Increased growth plate slope in a child with EFS [12].

1.2. Factors endocrine

Embrittlement of the upper femoral growth plate also appears to be related to endocrine factors. Three main hormones have been incriminated in the ethiopathogenesis of EFS. Growth hormone (GH), sex hormones and thyroid hormones.Harris [13] performed histological analyses on growth plate biopsies during EFS, he found alterations in the cell cycle and disorganizations of collagen under the influence of GH and sex hormones.The imbalance between GH and sex hormones changes the resistance of the growth plate. Indeed, under the influence of GH, the growth plate becomes hypertrophic. **The increase in its thickness leads to a decrease in its resistance.** Conversely, estrogens increase its resistance and accelerate its closure by slowing its activity [13]. This could explain the occurrence of EFS especially in the prepubertal period, during which GH is secreted in a pulsatile manner and precedes sex hormone secretion [14, 15]. Recent work published in 2017 by Halverson and colleagues [16] highlighted a possible involvement of leptin in the occurrence of EFS.

It has been demonstrated that between two adolescents of identical weight, the one who develops EFS has a significantly higher leptin level than the other. EFS can also be secondary to other conditions such as chronic renal failure and hypothyroidism. In a series published by Wilcox et al [17], hypothyroidism was noted in 25% of EFS, a decrease in testosterone levels in 76% of EFS and a decrease in GH levels in 87% of EFS. In a series of 131 EFS, Wells [18] noted a rate of 7% of endocrine pathologies and Mann [19] reported an endocrine abnormality in 4 of 20 children with EFS.

1.3. Factors genetic

A hereditary component has been suggested in some studies [20, 21]. Rennie et al [22] reported an incidence of 7-14% of cases with a family history of EFS. While Loder et al [23] estimated an incidence of EFS in a family of 39%. Genetic theory has also been suggested for the association of EFS with klinefelter syndrome or trisomy 21 [24]. Two EFS in two homozygous twins have been reported [25]. Some authors including Unsal [26] have incriminated the HLA DR4 haplotype as a contributing factor, while others, including Spero [25], have identified a link with HLA B12. To date, no gene has been identified as responsible for this condition.

1.4. Radiochemotherapy

It has been reported that EFS can be secondary to local irradiation [27]. A few rare cases occurring after local radiotherapy, alone or combined with chemotherapy, have been reported [28, 29].

2. Data from the literature and our series :

2.1. Prevalence

In a large worldwide multicenter series of 1630 children, the mean prevalence of epiphysiolysis was estimated to be 2/100,000 children. In the same series, this prevalence was variable according to race. Indeed, it was the lowest in Japanese and Indo-Mediterranean people and highest in Polynesian and black children who are 2-4 times more affected than white children [14]. The prevalence of EFS is higher in children with certain endocrine disorders such as sex hormone disorders, hypothyroidism, hyperparathyroidism and renal osteodystrophy [1,30]. Another more recent study published in 2018 confirmed that the incidence of EFS is variable across countries and ethnicities ranging from 0.2 per 100,000 children in eastern Japan to 10.8 per 100,000 children in the United States. This prevalence is clearly increasing and progresses with average body mass index (BMI) with age [30].

2.2. Gender

EFS affects boys more frequently than girls. In our series, 69.7% of the population studied were boys, i.e. a sex ratio of 2.3. This male predominance could be explained by: [1]

- The more pronounced turbulence of the boys.
- The difference in endocrine profile with later puberty in boys.

- A longer growth period with delayed growth plate fusion predisposing boys to a higher risk.

2.3. Age

EFS is a pathology of the adolescent between 9 and 16 years of age. It occurs at the onset of puberty during the phase of accelerated growth rate, with more than 60% of cases still having an open Y-shaped cartilage [31]. The average age of onset is 13 years and 6 months in boys and 12 years in girls [14]. In cases of EFS occurring in patients 10 years and younger or older than 16 years with an open physeal, an underlying endocrinopathy should be sought [32]. In our series, the mean age at diagnosis was 12.5 years with a standard deviation of 2 years and extremes of 9 and 16 years.

2.4. Obesity and morphotype

The review of the literature shows that overweight is the main risk factor for FES. It is common for this condition to be observed in children with an adiposogenic morphotype combining overweight and delayed pubertal development. A recent study in the United States by Maranho et al [33] that included 469 cases of EFS between 2000 and 2017 reported a BMI above the 95th percentile in 67% of cases.15% of children were overweight (85 ≤ BMI < 95th percentile) and those with normal weight (<85th percentile) accounted for only 18% of cases. The results we found are consistent with the literature. Indeed, in our study 58% of patients were obese and 13% were overweight. We also identified an association between obesity and bilateral form. In our series, among the 7 patients with a bilateral form, 5 were obese. We are in agreement with the literature regarding the role of obesity in the early occurrence of EFS. In our study, the children with an early form (age at diagnosis ≤ 10 years) were all obese.

2.5. Notion of trauma

The role of the trauma is variously appreciated according to the different studies. For many authors, it is a non-traumatic displacement constituting an accident at the end of growth and indicating premature aging of the growth plate. For others, EFS is described as occurring after a trauma in about 25% of cases [34]. However, although the hypothesis of a traumatic cause has been defended, the different studies have insisted for the last twenty years on the triggering or revealing role of the trauma, but not really the cause of the pathology. The onset of EFS may be caused by a sudden trauma or by a series of repetitive microtraumas that increase the shearing forces at the epiphysis, particularly when the thigh is abducted and laterally rotated [34,35].

Smida et al conducted a multicenter study involving 240 cases of EFS. They reported the notion of trauma in 43.5% of cases [1]. In our series, the history revealed the notion of trauma in 35.5% of cases. It was often minimal and generally occurred during a sporting activity.

2.6. Time to take charge

All studies conducted on EFS affirm that surgical management must be as urgent as possible in order to stop the progression of the displacement and avoid its increase. This reduces the risk of complications, the frequency of which increases with the extent of the displacement.Of the 83 hips treated, 80 were operated on within the first 24 hours of diagnosis. The average time between the first symptoms and the diagnosis was 2 months and 28 days. It is essential to emphasize the frequent delay in diagnosis, especially in chronic forms. This long duration of evolution characterizes the disease. It can be explained by the long tolerance of chronic and stable EFS on the one hand, and by the clinician's lack of awareness of the disease at the beginning of its course on the other.

3. Data clinical

3.1. Forms clinical
3.1.1. Classification according to the onset of the symptomatology

According to the time elapsed since the onset of the first symptoms, EFS are classified as chronic, acute and acute on chronic. This classification is based on the duration of the symptoms collected during questioning of the child and/or the parents. It has the advantage of describing the different forms encountered in clinical practice [36]. The incidence of the three forms is variously assessed across the series (Tables VI and VII).

Table VI: Frequency of the chronic form.

Author	Progressive revelation
Smida et al (2007) [1]	40,5%
Maranho et al (2019) [33]	54%
Our series	60%

Table VII: Frequency of acute and acute on chronic background forms.

Author	Acute form	Acute form on a chronic background
Smida et al (2007) [1]	19,3%	40,5%
Maranho et al (2019) [33]	29%	17%
Our series	23%	17%

3.1.2. Classification according to stability

Epiphysiolysis is classified as stable when there is no intra-articular effusion and walking with or without a cane is possible and as unstable when there is an intra-articular effusion and walking is impossible even with assistance. This classification is now the most widely used in clinical practice for its prognostic value: the frequency of occurrence of femoral osteonecrosis is strongly correlated with the stability of the epiphysis. Unstable EFS have a high risk of femoral osteonecrosis, which can be as high as 50% in some series, whereas in stable EFS the risk of necrosis is practically zero [3]. Stable EFS is the most frequent form in most studies (Table VIII).

Table VIII: Distribution of stable and unstable forms according to different series.

Author	Stable form	Unstable form
Loder (1993) [3]	54,5%	45,5%
Smida (2007) [1]	46%	54%
Maranho et al (2019) [33]	76%	24%
Our series	60%	40%

3.2. On the side reached

The predominance of left unilateral involvement in EFS is widely reported in the literature. The change from a static position (sitting or standing still) to a dynamic one (initiation of walking) may explain the more frequent occurrence of left EFS in right-handed patients who advance the right lower limb at the start of walking. It is the left lower limb that suffers the excessive mechanical constraints. Carlioz and Rey [10] reported that the left lower limb represents the limb of impulse and support in 70% of cases. In our series, left unilateral involvement was the most frequent with a rate of 59.2%.

3.3 Bilaterality

The prevalence of bilaterality varies according to the series. It ranges from 18 to 63 % [30]. Table IX below shows the rates o f bilateral involvement according to different series.

Table IX: Bilateral involvement.

Author	Bilateral involvement
Loder (1996) [14]	22,3%
Smida et al (2007) [1]	12%
Maranho et al (2019) [33]	10%
Our series	9%

4. Imaging

4.1. X-ray of the pelvis from face

Frontal radiographs of the pelvis can show evidence of slippage of the femoral epiphysis. Smida et al [1] found that Klein's line intersected the femoral epiphysis in 27% of cases, was tangent to the epiphysis in 41%, and passed outside the epiphysis in 31% of cases. Maranho et al [33] reported that Klein's line did not intersect the epiphysis in 85% of cases. In our series, the Klein line did not cut the epiphyseal core in 70% of cases. A Klein line cutting the epiphysis does not eliminate the diagnosis of EFS: case of pure posterior tilt.

4.2. Hip X-ray in profile; Incidence of Lauenstein

As soon as the diagnosis of EFS is evoked, the profile X-ray becomes essential to confirm the displacement and to assess its importance. It is often sufficient to make the diagnosis, especially in early forms with a small displacement that is difficult to detect on the frontal X-ray.

5. Treatment

5.1. Reduction before screwing

Reducing the slip prior to EFS surgery is a topic that has been widely discussed in the literature. Although reduction has been indicated by a few authors in acute forms, it was always proscribed in chronic forms. Some authors such as Gordon [37] and Jofe [38] have advocated orthopedic reduction only of the acute component of EFS. This reduction is achieved by flexion, abduction and internal rotation of the hip. It must be performed under anesthesia, on an orthopedic table and in a gentle manner. It allows closed reduction of the acute slip [39].

5.2. Means of fixation

5.3.1. Number of screws

Several studies have shown the efficacy of single screw fixation [5,14], but other authors have reported that in 20% of cases the slip progresses by an average of 10° after single screw fixation [40,41]. The number of screws required is related to the diameter used. For screws measuring **4.5 mm in diameter**, the cap is stabilized by **two screws** while a **single screw** of **6.0 or 7.0 mm** in diameter **is sufficient** to stabilize it.

5.3.2. Thread

Different types of threads are used.

> **Full thread cannulated screws**

They allow fixation and epiphysiodesis action such as the screw used by our team. (Cf. figure 5)

> **Distal threaded screw**

Miyanji [42] showed in an experimental study that there was no biomechanical superiority of full threading over partial threading (Figure 11). On the other hand, other studies [43, 44] found greater stability of the synthesis when using screws with full threads.

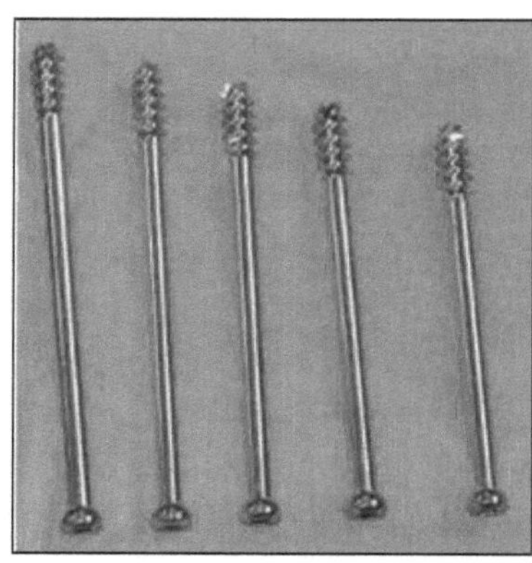

Figure 11: Screw with partial distal thread [45].

The purpose of this type of thread is to stop slippage by avoiding epiphysiodesis. Its designers [46] have shown that the smoothness of the distal part of the thread allows the femoral neck to continue to grow, while ensuring optimal fixation of the epiphysis with bone remodeling that can avoid complications related to architectural disorders (Figure 12).

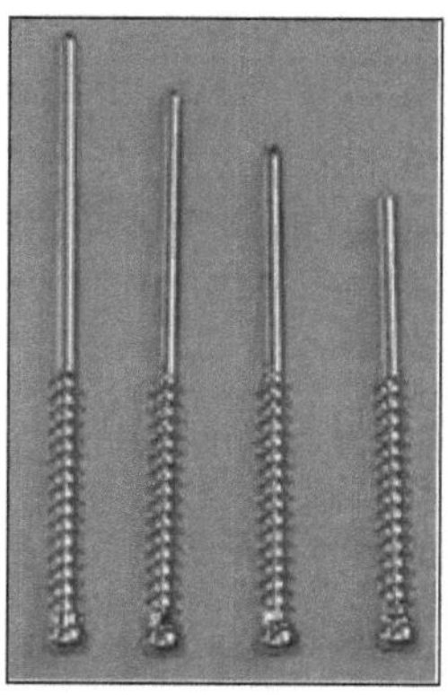

Figure 11: Screw with partial proximal thread [45].

> **Telescopic screws**

This type of screw was designed by Smida [1] (Figure 13) to achieve epiphyseal fixation while allowing the neck to grow. It is also used to avoid a frequent and little-known complication: coxa vara breva.

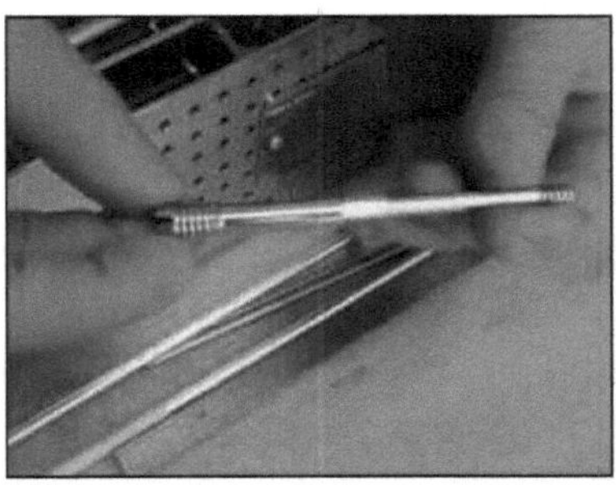

Figure 12: Telescopic screw.

In our series, fixation of the femoral epiphysis was done for all patients by a single full-thread cannulated screw measuring 7.0 mm in diameter with at least three turns of the coil holding the epiphyseal cap.

6. Follow-up / Progression of the slip after screwing

All patients who underwent EFS had a postoperative radio-clinical check-up at 6 weeks, 3 months, 6 months and 1 year of evolution, and then once a year in order to evaluate the functional results of the screw fixation, to look for signs of epiphysiodesis, to detect a possible complication and to monitor the contralateral hip joint In our series, only one case of significant progression of slippage (>5°) was noted. This complication is also very rarely found in series that have reported the results of EFS treatment by percutaneous screw fixation. Chen et al [47] reported only one case of worsening of slip after screw fixation in a series of 30 unstable EFS studied. The progression of slippage after percutaneous screw fixation has been explained in the literature by insufficient fixation. Some authors have reported that in 20% of cases, slip progresses by an average of 10° after fixation with a single screw [40,41]. Nevertheless, multiple screw fixation has not been shown to be superior, and the use of a single cannulated screw positioned in the middle of the epiphysis perpendicular to the physeal is the currently recommended technique of choice [48].

CONCLUSIONS

In order to understand the natural history of upper femoral epiphysiolysis (UFE), it seems fundamental to us to study its components, its evolution and its consequences. The ethiopathogenesis of FFE has not yet been elucidated, but several risk factors have been suggested. The main risk factor is overweight.The objectives of our work were to identify the biomechanical factors involved in the occurrence of upper femoral epiphysis through a case series and a review of the literature and to study the biomechanical factors of stability of the upper femoral epiphysis after percutaneous screw fixation allowing healing without sequelae.To meet these objectives, we conducted a retrospective, single-center, longitudinal study at the Béchir Hamza Children's Hospital in Tunis over a seven-year period. Eighty-three hips were treated for EFS by percutaneous screw fixation in seventy-six patients, including seven bilateral forms. We included EFS treated exclusively by percutaneous screw fixation with a postoperative follow-up of at least twelve months. In our study, we used three types of classification and a score.Seventy-six patients were divided into fifty-three boys (70%) and 23 girls (30%), with a sex ratio of 2.3. Age at surgery ranged from 9 to 16 years with an average of 12.5 years. Fifty-eight percent of the cases had a weight > +3 SD (Standard Deviations) with 11% having an adiposogenic morphotype. 13% of the cases had a weight between +2 and +3 SD and 29% had a normal weight. The delay between the EFS diagnosis and surgical management did not exceed 24 hours for 98% of patients. The stable form represented 60% and the unstable form 40% of the cases. For the eighty-three hips studied, we obtained 47% stage I, 43% stage II and 10% stage III. For epiphyseal fixation, we used a Veet-Woot type screw with a washer. We evaluated the results of the screw fixation based on the Postel and Merle d'Aubigné (PMA) grading. At an average follow-up of 5.66 years, we obtained excellent results in 56.6% of cases, good results in 36.1%, fair results in 4.8%, and poor results in 2.4% of cases.Comparing our results with those of the literature, the mechanical factor represents the main risk factor for EFS. Obesity was considered a risk factor by all the series studied. It results in the decrease of femoral anteversion and increased shear forces. Still in favor of a mechanical explanation, it has been shown that the risk of epiphysiolysis was greater in children with a greater slope of the upper femoral growth plate Other metabolic factors have been incriminated such as hypothyroidism, growth hormone deficiency, chronic renal failure. Genetic factors have also been implicated in the genesis of EFS, such as trisomy 21 and ethnicity. Secondary EFS has also been reported in cancer patients undergoing chemo-radiotherapy. The common denominator between all these risk factors is the decreased biomechanical strength of the subcapital growth plate and its perichondral rim. Percutaneous screw fixation, with or without reduction, is the gold standard for the management of small and medium displacement PSA. Its objective is to stabilize the femoral cap, thereby stopping and worsening the slippage. Several types of devices and implants are available on the market, but we recommend the Weet-voot cannulated and threaded 7mm diameter screw. The positioning of the screw in the cap is also a major factor in stability. The screw should be in the center of the cap on the front and side x-rays. At least three turns of the screw to hold the cap in place and six weeks of unloading of the operated hip are also biomechanical requirements for the stability of the epiphyseal cap. Our results at the last recoil are consistent with those in the literature.Our work opens the horizons for a thesis in the field of biomechanics engineering applied to the musculoskeletal system allowing a laboratory study to better identify the elements of postoperative stability.

REFERENCES

1. Smida. M, Ben Ghachem. M, Bouchoucha. S. Superior femoral epiphysiolysis. XXIII National Congress of the SOTCOT. 2007. p10 https://www.fichier-pdf.fr/2014/03/16/epiphysiolyse-femorale-superieure-sotcot

2. Fahey JJ, O'Brien ET. Acute slipped capital femoral epiphysis. Review of the literature and report of ten cases. J Bone Joint Surg Am. 1965;47:1105-27.

3. Loder R, Richards BS, Shapiro PS, Reznick LR, Aronso DD. Acute slipped capital femoral epiphysis: The importance of physeal stability. J Bone Joint Surg Am. 1993;75:1134-40.

4. Kallio PE, Paterson DC, Foster BK, Lequesne GW. Classification in slipped capital femoral epiphysis. Sonographic assessment of stability and remodeling. Clin Orthop Relat Res. 1993;294:196-203.

5. Southwick WO. Osteotomy through the lesser trochanter for slipped capital femoral epiphysis. J Bone Joint Surg Am. 1967;49(5):807-35.

6. Merle d'Aubigné RM, Postel M. Function al results of hip arthroplasty with acrylic prosthesis. J Bone Joint Surg Am. 1954;36:451-75.

7. Pritchett JW, Perdue KD. Mechanical factors in slipped capital femoral epiphysis. J Pediatr Orthop. 1988;8(4):385-8.

8. Gelberman RH, Cohen MS, Shaw BA, Kasser JR, Griffin PP, Wilkinson RH. The association of femoral retroversion with slipped capital femoral epiphysis. J Bone Joint Surg Am. 1986;68(7):1000-7.

9. Galbraith RT, Gelberman RH, Hajek PC, Baker LA, Sartoris DJ, Rab GT, et al. Obesity and decreased femoral anteversion in adolescence. J Orthop Res. 1987;5(4):523-8.

10. Carlioz H, Pous JG, Rey JC. Upper femoral epiphysiolysis. Rev Chir Orthop Reparatrice Appar Mot. 1968;54(5):387-491.

11. Jacquemier M, Noca P, Dick R, Bollini G, Moulia-Pelat JP, Migliani R, et al. Study of femoral anteversion in adolescent upper femoral epiphysiolysis. About 25 cases. Rev Chir Orthop Reparatrice Appar Mot. 1991;77(8):530-6.

12. Abu Amara S, Leroux J, Lechevallier J. Surgery for slipped capital femoral epiphysis in adolescents. Orthop Traumatol Surg Res. 2014;100(1 Suppl):S157-67.

13. Harris Wr. The endocrine basis for slipping of the upper femoral epiphysis. J Bone Joint Surg Am. 1950;2;32-B(1):5-11.
14. Loder RT. The demographics of slipped capital femoral epiphysis. An international multicenter study. Clin Orthop Relat Res. 1996;(322):8-27.
15. Exner GU. Growth and pubertal development in slipped capital femoral epiphysis: a longitudinal study. J Pediatr Orthop. 1986;6(4):4039.
16. Halverson SJ, Warhoover T, Mencio GA, Lovejoy SA, Martus JE, Schoenecker JG. Leptin elevation as a risk factor for slipped capital femoral epiphysis independent of obesity status. J Bone Joint Surg Am. 2017;99(10):865-872.
17. Wilcox PG, Weiner DS, Leighley B. Maturation factors in slipped capital femoral epiphysis. J Pediatr Orthop. 1988;8(2):196-200.
18. Wells D, King JD, Roe TF, Kaufman FR. Review of slipped capital femoral epiphysis associated with endocrine disease. J Pediatr Orthop. 1993;13(5):610-4.

19. Mann DC, Weddington J, Richton S. Hormonal studies in patients with slipped capital femoral epiphysis without evidence of endocrinopathy. J Pediatr Orthop. 1988;8(5):543-5.
20. Hägglund G, Hansson LI, Sandström S. Familial slipped capital femoral epiphysis. Acta Orthop Scand. 1986;57(6):510-2.

21. Mayrargue E, Hamel A, Le Cour Grandmaison F, Guillard S, Rogez JM. A case report A familial form of epiphyseal slippage. Arch Ped. 2008;15(5):1029.
22. Rennie AM. The inheritance of slipped upper femoral epiphysis. J Bone Joint Surg Br. 1982;64(2):180-4.
23. Loder RT, Nechleba J, Sanders JO, Doyle P. Idiopathic slipped capital femoral epiphysis in Amish children. J Bone Joint Surg Am. 2005;87(3):543-9.
24. Diwan A, Diamond T, Clarke R, Patel MK, Murrell GA, Sekel R. Familial slipped capital femoral epiphysis: a report and considerations in management. Aust N Z J Surg. 1998;68(9):647-9.
25. Spero CR, Masciale JP, Tornetta P, Star MJ, Tucci JJ. Slipped capital femoral epiphysis in black children: incidence of chondrolysis. J Pediatr Orthop. 1992;12(4):444-8.
26. Unsal E, Gülay Z, Günal I. The association of HLA-DR4 antigen with juvenile chronic arthritis and slipped capital femoral epiphysis. Arch Orthop Trauma Surg. 2001;121(10):571-3.

27. Loder RT, Hensinger RN, Alburger PD, Aronsson DD, Beaty JH, Roy DR, et al. Slipped capital femoral epiphysis associated with radiation therapy. J Pediatr Orthop. 1998;18(5):630-6.

28. Mainard-Simard L, Journeau P. Epiphysiolysis of the hip. Feuil Radiol. 2014;54:292- 303.

29. Liu SC, Tsai CC, Huang CH. Atypical slipped capital femoral epiphysis after radiotherapy and chemotherapy. Clin Orthop Relat Res. 2004;(426):212-8.

30. Mainard-Simard L. Epiphysiolysis of the hip. Feuil Radiol. 2018; 13(4):1-10.

31. Puylaert D, Dimeglio A, Bentahar T. Staging puberty in slipped capital femoral epiphysis: importance of the triradiate cartilage. J Pediatr Orthop. 2004;24(2):144-7.

32. Loder RT, Wittenberg B, DeSilva G. Slipped capital femoral epiphysis associated with endocrine disorders. J Pediatr Orthop. 1995;15(3):349-56.

33. Maranho DA, Bixby S, Miller PE, Novais EN. A novel classification system for slipped capital femoral epiphysis based on the radiographic relationship of the epiphyseal tubercle and the metaphyseal socket. J Bone Joint Surg. 2019;4(4):e0033.

34. Witzel K, Raschka C. Epiphysiolysis capitis femoris caused by a repeat minor trauma. MMW Fortschr Med. 2005;147(16):41-3.

35. Moore LK, Dally AF. Medical Anatomy: Fundamental Aspects and Clinical Application. Editions de Boeck. 2006;p510.

36. Klein C, Odent T, Glorion C. Superior femoral epiphysiolysis. EMC App Locom. 2016;14-321-A-21

37. Gordon JE, Abrahams MS, Dobbs MB, Luhmann SJ, Schoenecker PL. Early reduction, arthrotomy, and cannulated screw fixation in unstable slipped capital femoral epiphysis treatment. J Pediatr Orthop. 2002;22(3):352-8.

38. Jofe MH, Lehman W, Ehrlich MG. Chondrolysis following slipped capital femoral epiphysis. J Pediatr Orthop B. 2004;13(1):29-31.

39. Boero S, Brunenghi GM, Carbone M, Stella G, Calevo MG. Pinning in slipped capital femoral epiphysis: long-term follow-up study. J Pediatr Orthop B. 2003;12(6):372-9.

40. Denton JR. Fixation with a single screw for slipped capital femoral

epiphysis. J Bone Joint Surg Am. 1993;75(3):469.

41. Aronson DD, Carlson WE. Slipped capital femoral epiphysis. A prospective study of fixation with a single screw. J Bone Joint Surg Am. 1992;74(6):810-9.

42. Miyanji F, Mahar A, Oka R, Pring M, Wenger D. Biomechanical comparison of fully and partially threaded screws for fixation of slipped capital femoral epiphysis. J Pediatr Orthop. 2008;28(1):49-52.

43. Upasani V, Kishan S, Oka R, Mahar A, Rohmiller M, Pring M, et al. Biomechanical analysis of single screw fixation for slipped capital femoral epiphysis: are more threads across the physis necessary for stability? J Pediatr Orthop. 2006;26(4):474-8.

44. Dragoni M, Heiner AD, Costa S, Gabrielli A, Weinstein SL. Biomechanical study of 16-mm threaded, 32-mm threaded, and fully threaded SCFE screw fixation. J Pediatr Orthop. 2012;32(1):70-4.

45. Abu Amara S, Leroux J, Lechevallier J. Surgery for slipped capital femoral epiphysis in adolescents. Orthop Traumatol Surg Res. 2014;100(1 Suppl):S157-67.

46. Sailhan F, Courvoisier A, Brunet O, Chotel F, Berard J. Continued growth of the hip after fixation of slipped capital femoral epiphysis using a single cannulated screw with a proximal threading. J Child Orthop. 2011;5(2):83-8.

47. Chen RC, Schoenecker PL, Dobbs MB, Luhmann SJ, Szymanski DA, Gordon JE. Urgent reduction, fixation, and arthrotomy for unstable slipped capital femoral epiphysis J Pediatr Orthop. 2009;29(7):687-94.

48. Klein C, Haraux E, Leroux J, Gouron R. Superior femoral epiphysiolysis. Arch Pediatr. 2017;24(3):301-5.

ANNEXES

Appendix 1: Fahey and O'Brien classification [2].

This is the oldest classification, but it is still relevant. Fahey and O'Brien classify EFS according to the duration of symptoms.
- **Chronic form:** EFS is considered chronic when the pain has been present for more than 3 weeks. The intensity of the pain is often moderate.

- **Acute form:** An EFS is considered acute when the pain has been evolving for less than 3 weeks. The pain is intense, the functional impotence is sometimes total.

- **Acute on chronic form:** An acute on chronic EFS is characterized by an exacerbation of the pain due to an acute slip occurring on a chronic painful background.

Appendix 2: Loder and Kallio Classification

Currently, the clinical and radiological classification taking into account the stability of the epiphysis is the most used to guide the therapeutic indications and seems to be the best correlated to the prognosis.

Clinically, stability depends on the ability to walk:[6]

- an unstable slip is characterized by the impossibility of walking, even with of the canes, regardless of the age of the symptoms.

- a slip is stable when walking and supporting are possible with or without canes.

At the imaging level, stability depends on the existence of an intra-articular effusion. [7]

If the ultrasound shows an intra-articular effusion, the EFS is considered unstable. If there is no intra-articular effusion, the epiphysiolysis is described as stable EFS.

Appendix 3: Radiographic classification based on Southwick angle measurement [5].

It is based on the measurement of the Southwick angle on the profile film. This angle is formed between the axis of the cervix and the line perpendicular to the axis of the cervical cartilage. It allows to define three stages according to the severity:

- **Stage I**: Corresponds to a tilt angle < 30°; low slip
- **Stage II:** Corresponds to an angle between 30° and 60°; moderate slippage

- **Stage III:** Corresponds to an angle > 60°; severe slippage.

Appendix 4: Postel and Merle d'Aubigné (PMA) scoring [6].

		Pain	Mobility	Walk
			No vicious attitude : only take into account the amplitude in flexion	
6		No	Vicious attitude: remove 1 point for 20° or more of irreducible flexion or external rotation and 2 points for 10°. or + of irreducible abduction, adduction, internal rotation Amplitude in flexion ≥ 90°	Perfect stability Normal and Unlimited operation
5		Rare and light, not preventing normal activity	Flexion amplitude 75 to 85°.	Imperfect stability Slight lameness with fatigue Cane sometimes for long distances
4		Compatible with reduced physical activity, allowing 1/2hour or more of walking	Amplitude in flexion 55 to 70°.	Slight instability Clear lameness Often a cane to go out
3		Stopping the walk after 20 minutes	Amplitude in flexion 35 to 50°.	Instability Strong lameness A cane in permanence
2		Stopping the walk after 10 minutes	Flexion amplitude < 30	High instability 2 canes, 1 cane-crutch sometimes
1		Very keen to mobilize and support, do allowing only a few steps	Reduced flexion + important vicious attitude	Monopodal support not possible 2 crutches or cane-crutches
0		Very lively and permanent, not allowing walking, confining the patient to bed and causing insomnia	Reduced flexion + important vicious attitude	Standing not possible Support not possible Grabber

Appraisals based on total points:

Total points	Result
18	Excellent
15-17	Good
12-14	Medium
<12	Bad

BIOMECHANICS OF SLIPPED CAPITAL FEMORAL EPIPHYSIS IN ADOLESCENTS: RISK FACTORS AND STABILITY CRITERIA

Abstract

Background:
The etiopathogenesis of slipped capital femoral epiphysis (SCFE) is not yet understood, but several risk factors have been suggested. The common denominator between all the risk factors is the decrease in the biomechanical resistance of the growth cartilage under capital and its perichondral ring.
The objectives were to identify the biomechanical factors involved in the occurrence of upper femoral epiphysis through a series of cases and a review of the literature and to study the biomechanical factors of stability of the upper femoral epiphysis after percutaneous screwing allowing healing without sequelae.

Methods:
Statistical analysis of the data was performed using SPSS. The results were evaluated clinical by the PMA score and radiological by the calculation of the residual tilt angle.

Results:
The main biomechanical factor involved in the occurrence of SCFE was obesity. It was identified in 58% of cases with an adipose-genital morphotype which represented 11%. The second factor was hormonal disturbances with an age of onset of 9 years. Biomechanical factors for screwing stability were screw diameter and thread type, all of our screws were 7mm full thread diameter. The second factor was the centering of the screw and the number of turns that hold the epiphyseal cap. We noted only one case of sliding progression after screwing. The third factor was the prohibition of postoperative support for 6 weeks for all of our patients. The overall result was excellent to good.

Conclusion:
The identification of the biomechanical factors involved in the genesis of SCFE allows prophylactic pinning for the healthy hip. Knowledge of biomechanical factors during the placement of the cephalic screw is the guarantee of a stable osteosynthesis.

Key-words: Biomechanics, Musculoskeletal system, Slipped capital femoral epiphysis, Percutaneous pinning

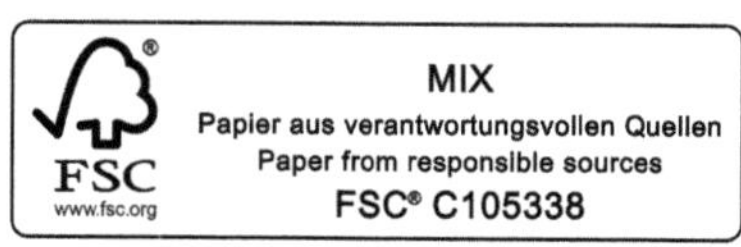

Printed by Books on Demand GmbH, Norderstedt / Germany